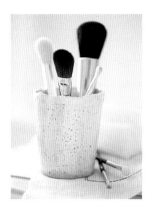

blissful beauty
MORNING NOON & NIGHT

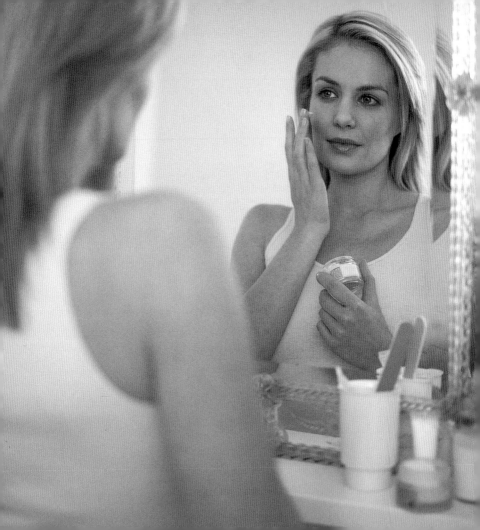

LIZ WILDE

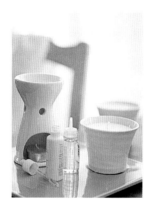

blissful beauty
MORNING NOON & NIGHT

RYLAND
PETERS
& SMALL

LONDON NEW YORK

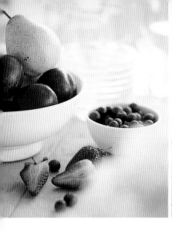
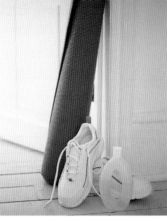
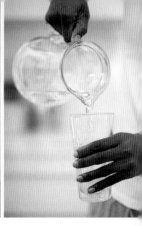

Senior Designer Megan Smith
Senior Editor Clare Double
Picture Researcher Emily Westlake
Production Gemma Moules
Art Director Anne-Marie Bulat
Publishing Director Alison Starling

First published in the
United Kingdom in 2007
by Ryland Peters & Small
20–21 Jockey's Fields
London WC1R 4BW
www.rylandpeters.com

Text, design and photographs
© Ryland Peters & Small 2007
10 9 8 7 6 5 4 3 2 1

Printed and bound in China

ISBN: 978-1-84597-400-8

A CIP record for this book is available
from the British Library.

If you are in any doubt about your
health, please consult your doctor
before making any changes to your
usual dietary and well-being regime.
Essential oils are very powerful and
potentially toxic if used too liberally.
Please follow the guidelines and never
use the oils neat on bare skin, unless
advised otherwise. This book is not
suitable for anyone during pregnancy.

Acknowledgments
The author would like to thank all
her wonderful friends and family.
Visit Liz Wilde's website at
www.wildelifecoaching.com
to subscribe to her free Monthly
Motivator Mail.

contents

Introduction

DO YOU SPEND YOUR DAYS coping with what life throws at you and congratulating yourself every evening that once again you've almost succeeded in keeping your friends, family and employers happy? That's worth celebrating, except for the fact that somewhere in this delicate balance is your need to be happy too. Happiness is not an accident. Your energy, enthusiasm and self-esteem are constantly under threat and if you don't practise simple techniques every day to renew them, these parts of you will get lost in the busyness of life.

You may be thinking that you haven't got time for yourself in your already frantic day, which is why all the habits in this book are quick and simple to do. Little things make a big difference, and small changes are not only easier to make but require no discipline at all.

Do something to make you feel good every day and it becomes a habit you're likely to continue for a very long time.

We are what we repeatedly do.
Excellence, then, is not an act
but a habit. ARISTOTLE

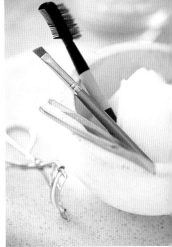

Not only will feel-good habits lift you out of a bad
mood, they'll also significantly improve your
quality of life, not to mention your health and
well-being. Link your habit to a regular part of
your routine (tea break, commuting, bedtime) and
you'll also have a better chance of remembering.
Forgotten yourself during a particularly hectic day?
No problem, just make a conscious choice to do
something you love tomorrow.

Enjoy fitting these habits into your day. There's
nothing more important in your life than happiness,
yet it's only possible to live happily ever after one
day at a time. And as every woman knows, taking
joy in life is nature's very best cosmetic.

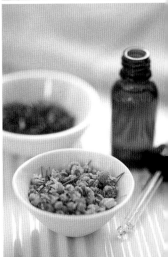

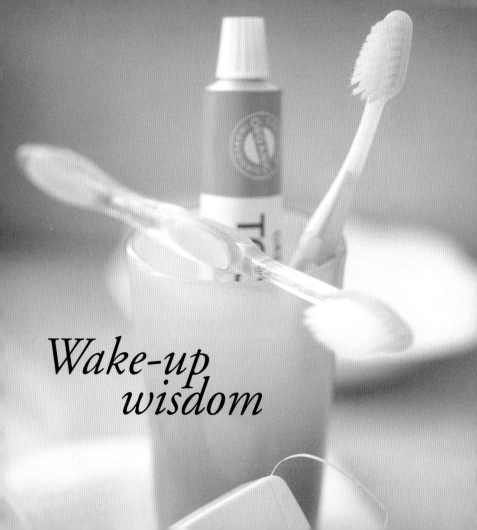

Wake-up wisdom

wear more cashmere

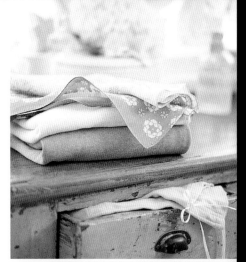

RESEARCH SHOWS that feeling attractive to others significantly boosts our mood, not to mention our self-esteem. So what are you saving your best self for? Wear clothes, shoes, underwear and fragrance you love every day. Choose outfits that fit and flatter your body (rather than the body you'd like to have), and fabrics that feel good against your skin. Simply showing this much affection to yourself at the beginning of your day will give you a head start on the potential chaos ahead.

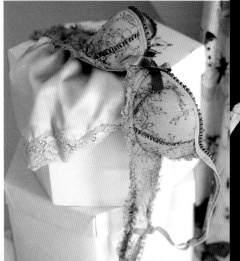

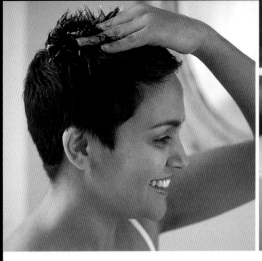
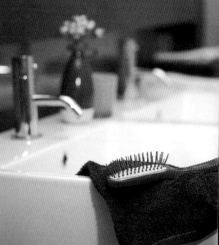

bad morning hair fixes

* When there's no time to style your hair from scratch, simply wash and blow-dry your fringe, which will make everything feel so much fresher.

* Absorb excess oil from three-day-old roots by rubbing in a little talcum powder, which will also add volume, or simply use blotting paper.

* Last night's pub smell can be erased in seconds by lightly misting your hair with fabric freshener.

* Flat hair can be bulked up instantly by hanging your head upside-down and spritzing the roots with hairspray. Let it dry for two seconds before flicking your hair back.

* Smooth frizz with a dollop of serum rubbed between your palms and smoothed over the surface of your hair.

* For a quick up-do that's posher than your gym ponytail, take sections of the tail, wind around your finger, and grip in place, leaving the ends free.

making up for anything

* Put make-up on bare skin and you can expect it to be gone in an hour. Instead, first apply foundation. Use your fingers, as they press the product into your skin so it stays put much longer – and you'll need to use much less.

* A loose powder over foundation will stop it evaporating, and absorb T-zone oil and perspiration all day. Use an eyeshadow brush to dust over lids for all-day smudge-free shadow, but avoid cheeks to keep a flattering gleam.

* For flake-free mascara, separate lashes between each coat (when dry) with a lash comb. A waterproof or water-resistant product will always last longer, and go easy with moisturizer under the eyes, which will encourage make-up to move.

* Waxy pencils on warm eyelids will melt and move. Instead, line your eyes with a powder shadow using a wet brush and the result will last ten times longer.

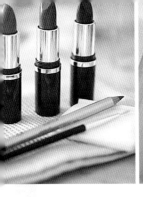 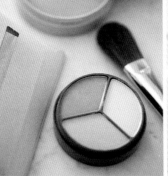 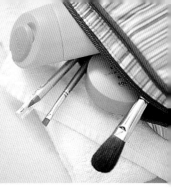

* For long-lasting eyes, choose cream-to-powder products that contain silicones. They slide on easily but set the moment they come into contact with your skin's warmth. Or set cream shadows with a little translucent powder applied with an eyeshadow brush.

* Test a lipstick's staying power before buying by applying a small amount to the palm of your hand. Leave for three minutes, wipe off with a tissue and you should be left with a tint on your skin.

* No lipstick, however long-lasting, will stick around unless you apply it to clean, dry lips. For extra longevity, use a lip liner all over lips as a base to give your lipstick something to grab on to.

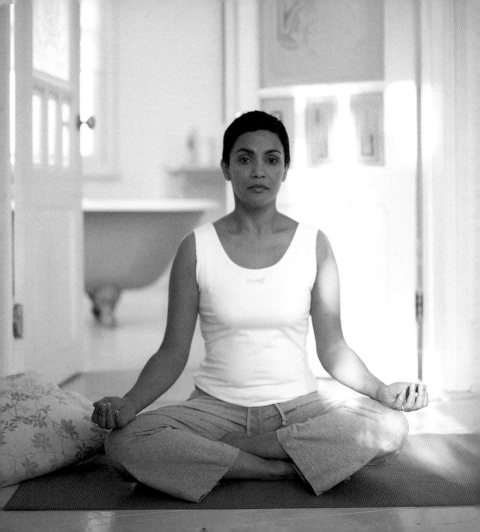

bathroom yoga

WATCH ANY SLUMBERING cat or dog. The first thing they do on waking is enjoy a luxurious stretch. Flexibility keeps your body healthy and you can practise yoga's two basic poses – a downward- and an upward-facing dog – at your bathroom sink without having to invest in a yoga mat.

* Stand about three feet away from your sink with feet hip-width apart and facing forward. With legs straight, bend forward from the waist and hold onto the sink. Look up slightly and draw your bottom away from the sink to stretch out your spine. Hold for five deep breaths.

* Stand up straight and step a little closer to the sink. Now push down on the sink with straight arms and bring your hips forward so you rise up on your toes. Keep your shoulders relaxed and look to the edge of the ceiling. Feel a gentle stretch in your back as you breathe deeply five times.

5 running-late shortcuts

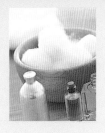

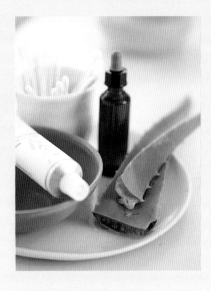

✳ Last-minute manicure? Dip still-tacky nails in a bowl of ice-cold water for a few minutes to set them hard.

✳ Chew fennel seeds. They not only freshen your breath, but also help with digestion after bolting down your breakfast.

✳ For sensitive-skin mornings, soak a cotton wool ball in a mixture of aloe vera and water and gently wipe over your face. Or wake up tired skin fast by leaving skincare products in the fridge overnight.

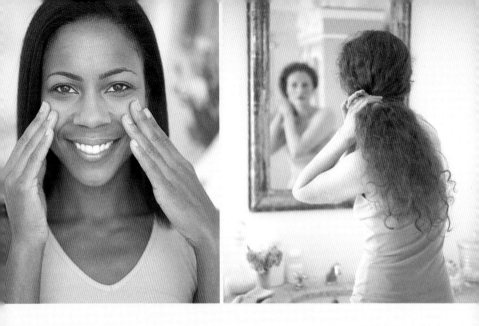

✳ No time for cucumber slices? Gently massage either side of your nose to release fluid retention and reduce puffiness around your eyes.

✳ If your curly hair turns to frizz overnight, sleep with a silk scarf tied loosely around your head. This will cut down friction during the night – and styling time first thing.

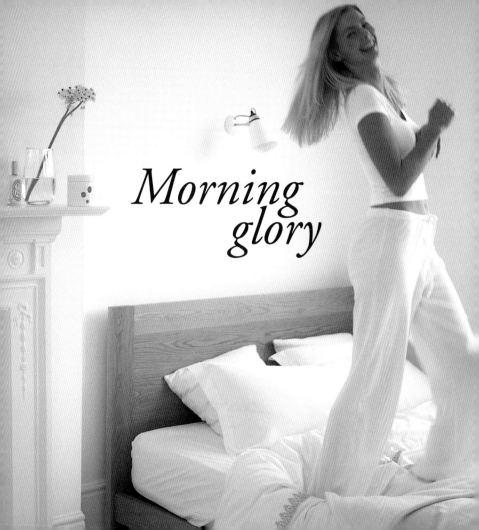

Morning glory

walk happy

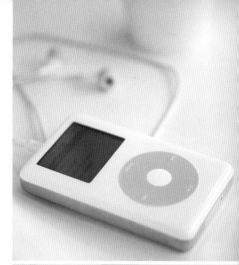

HAPPY WALKING works the same way as smiling when you're down. Your feelings don't take long to catch up. That's because body movements affect our thinking patterns, which means that if you walk like a happy person you'll begin to think happy thoughts, too. So do what it takes to put a spring in your step. Compile upbeat playlists on your iPod, visualize yourself doing something exciting, or simply pretend you're in a feel-good movie. You won't just be cheering your mind, you'll be slimming your hips – stride out with arms swinging and you increase calories burned by almost 50%, too.

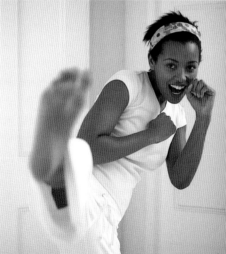

the fragrance factor

THE RIGHT FRAGRANCE can recreate intense memories from the past, because we respond to smell emotionally. Think back to the perfume your mother wore when you were young (easier still, ask her) or the scent you sprayed before hitting the town on teenage nights out. Visit the beauty hall in your local department store for inspiration on how to relive your favourite moments in life. And don't let scent snobs put you off buying something less than designer – the bottle (and advertising) are the most expensive part of any premium-brand perfume. If you have no scents in your memory bank, start creating your own pleasure perfumes. Wear a fragrance every day on holiday, and you'll always associate it with relaxing times. Or use the same scent on nights out, so the minute you spray it on you'll feel uplifted (even if you're only travelling to work on the bus).

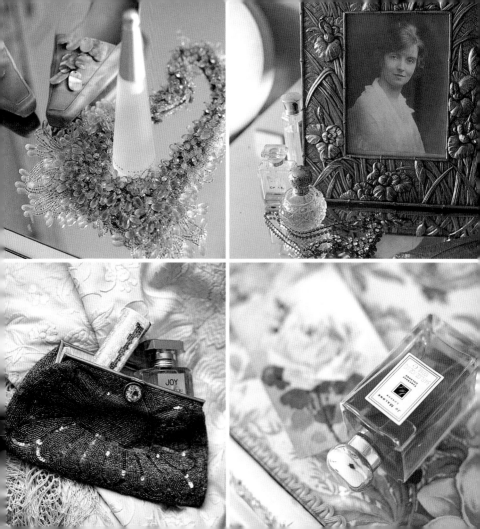

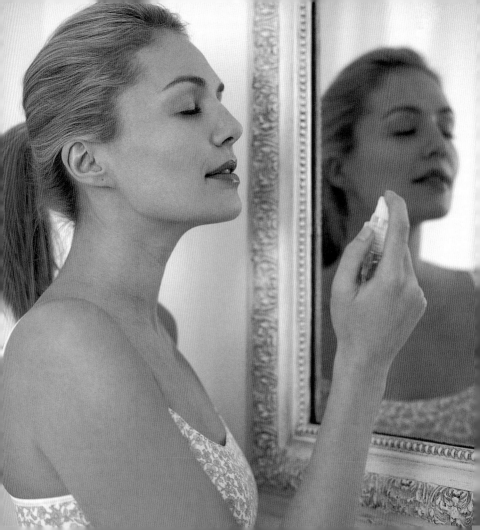

grooming on the go

* After you've eaten your mid-morning orange, rub the white pith against your teeth for a natural whitening shine.

* Prevent reapplied lipstick transferring to your teeth by popping your index finger in your mouth and then pulling it out. Any excess colour on the inside of your lips will come off on your finger, not on your teeth 30 minutes later.

* To wipe away smudges without rubbing, use a cotton bud dipped in moisturizer, then clean up with the other end.

* Spritz your face with water to soften make-up that's gone cakey. To control shine, spray with rose water and then lightly blot with a tissue.

* Apply lip colour with an eyeshadow brush, which not only makes the job quicker and easier but also gives you far more control over colour intensity than a tiny lip brush.

YOU'RE FAR MORE LIKELY to feel happy if you have a sense of control over your life. The simplest way to achieve this is to set up what you want to happen. The next time you're in an out-of-your-control situation (for example staying with your in-laws), think about what *is* within your control (enjoying long walks in the countryside, savouring home-made cooking and so on). Your intention need not even be directly related to what you're doing. Pick a boring activity such as walking to the station in the morning and choose your intention: to notice beautiful things around you, to smile at everyone you see… It can even make something you do without thinking every day start to feel like the highlight of your day.

set your intention

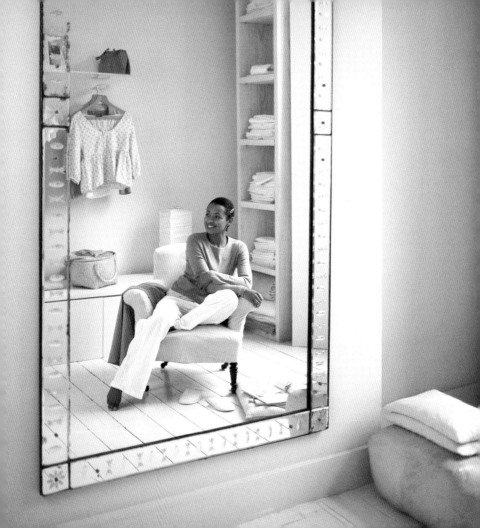

5 ways
to feel fresh
at work

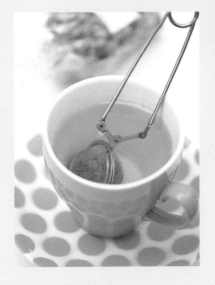

✳ Boss driving you mad? Rather than focusing on their bad points (indecisive, irrational), write a list of their good ones (supportive, approachable). Keep it handy for those moments when you're tempted to act in a way you might regret. After all, to gain respect, first you have to show it.

✳ Our brains love order and achieving makes us feel good, so when morale's low make a daily to-do list. Too long a list? Then prioritize everything into very important, important, and not so important. Knowing the difference will save you valuable time and energy.

✳ Get fresh air whenever possible by opening a window or taking a 10-minute tea break outside. Sunlight is another proven mood improver, so never work through a sunny lunchtime.

✳ Get into the habit of checking your personal speed. What gear are you in? Comfortable, fast or supersonic? Slow yourself down by doing everything at a calmer pace. Talk slower, move slower and breathe slower.

✳ Work in short spurts, taking frequent mini-breaks to stretch your neck, roll your shoulders and relax your eyes. If your job's boring, break the day into small sections, giving yourself something different to think about for each one.

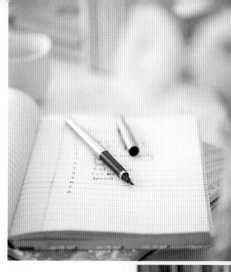

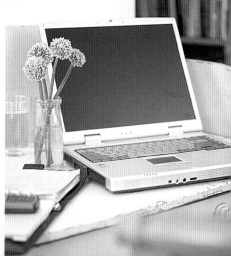

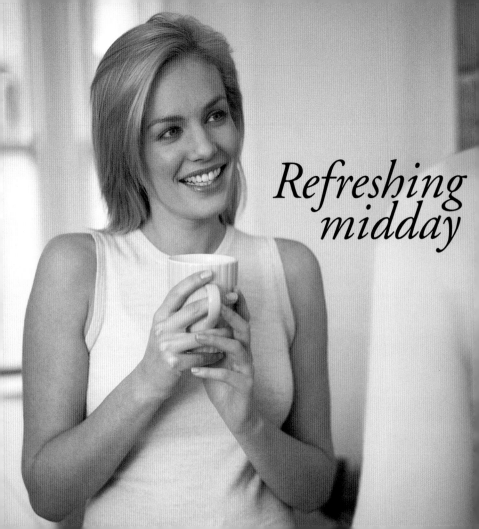

Refreshing midday

happiness hit list

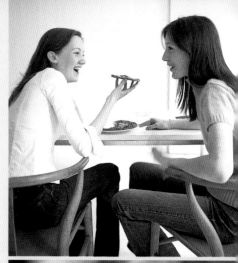

FEELING GOOD is not an accident. If you genuinely want to be happy, you must focus on what will get you there. Spend a lunch hour writing a list of all the things you love doing, from talking with laugh-out-loud friends to crying over an old film, from walking your dog along the river to curling up on the sofa with a good book. Making a list forces you to take responsibility for your happiness, rather than just hoping good things will happen. Then put your list somewhere visible and promise yourself at least one love-life activity every day.

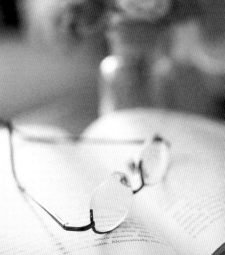

soft-focus walking

SLOW DOWN your thoughts and it's surprising what insights come into your head. A walk outside is the perfect way to clear the clutter. Switch to intuition mode and you could shift your perception, too.

* Choose somewhere quiet (you might feel a little disorientated, so steer clear of busy roads!) and pick a problem from your busy morning to mull over.

* As you walk, focus somewhere in the middle distance. Allow your eyes to go soft as if you're looking at one of those hidden images in 3-D pictures.

* Notice that, at some point, the world appears to be moving towards you, rather than you moving to it.

* Keep your eyes unfocused for as long as possible and allow your mind to wander. You may well be surprised where it goes…

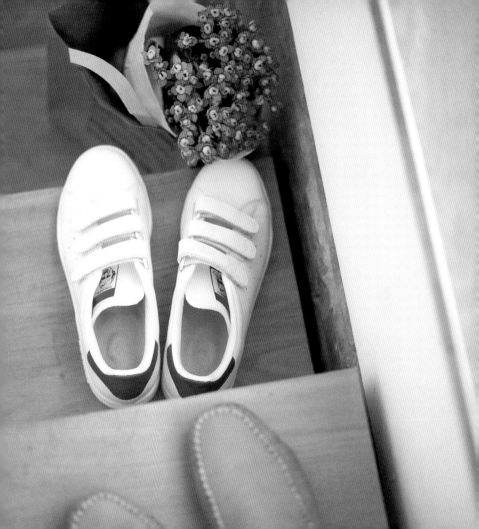

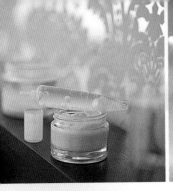
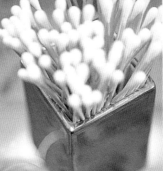
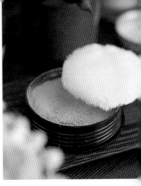

fast look-good fixes

* Add instant radiance to your skin by blending a little pink or peach cream blusher over the apples of your cheeks, then dab what's left on your fingertips over temples and tip of your chin.

* Lighten up any dark, shadowy areas – the sides of your nose, between your eyes, the outer corners of your eyes and under your lower lip – with a light-reflecting concealer pen.

* Rather than reapply mascara all over, just add a second coat at the outer corners of your upper lashes (wiggle the brush from side to side to avoid clumping) to make your eyes look bigger.

* Beware using a concealer one shade lighter than your skin to cover a spot, as this will only draw attention to the area. Instead, use a brush to apply a foundation that exactly matches your skin tone directly onto the blemish and blend.

* If you're having an off-day, get a blow-dry in your lunch hour. It's cheaper than a massage and will make you look and feel 100% better.

* For an instant face-lift effect, apply a small amount of a base that's slightly lighter than your usual one just down the centre of your face and blend.

* To hide grey roots around your hairline, apply a powder eyeshadow in a similar shade to your hair colour with a cotton bud or old toothbrush.

* A sweep of sand-coloured eyeshadow will make tired eyes look less red.

* Rub a little lip balm between finger and thumb and pat onto cheekbones for a healthy, youthful glow.

5 tricks to take the frown off your face

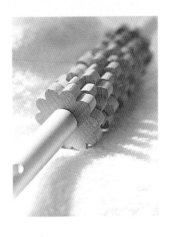

✳ Direct your mind to what's good in your life by asking the right questions. Ask yourself: What's going well for me right now? What have I got to look forward to? It really is that easy to change your perspective.

✳ Your breathing changes with your mood, and luckily it works the other way round too. Breathing in a deep, relaxed way is the fastest way to dissolve a bad mood in minutes.

✳ Change your shoes at lunchtime (especially if you've been standing or walking all morning) and your whole body will feel refreshed. Or keep a foot roller in your drawer to massage away midday aches and pains.

✳ A power nap in the middle of the day will keep you going for the next six hours. You don't even need to close your eyes (although do so if you can). Just sit quietly, breathe slowly and think relaxing thoughts. Even five minutes of deep rest will set you up for the afternoon ahead.

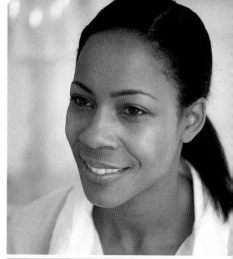

✳ If your neck feels stiff, gently walk your thumb and fingers across the ball of your foot below your toes and then around the base of your big toe. For an aching back, walk your thumb down the inner edge of your foot, following the bones along the arch.

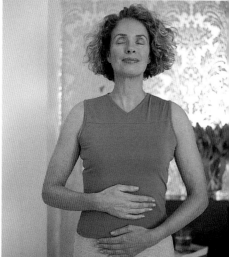

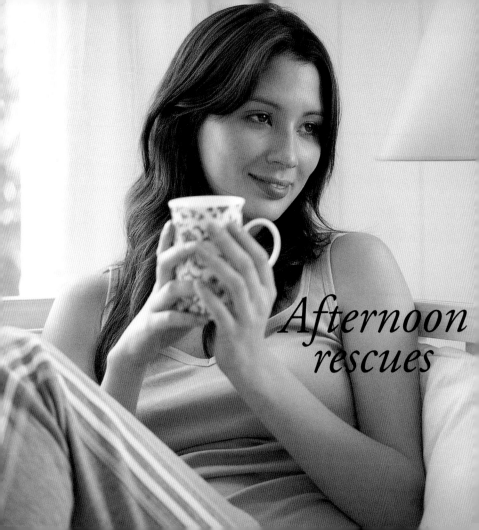

Afternoon rescues

say it with a smile

SMILING USES FACIAL MUSCLES
linked to areas in your brain that
produce feelings of joy. And not only
does smiling make you feel happier, it
puts the person you're smiling at in a
better mood, too. A sincere smile makes
you more likeable, and a smile that
shows in both eyes and mouth has even
more power. Nothing to smile about?
Forcing one causes a response in your
brain that actually produces genuine
positive emotions, and the more you
strengthen your smile muscles, the
more smiley your face will be –
whatever your mood.

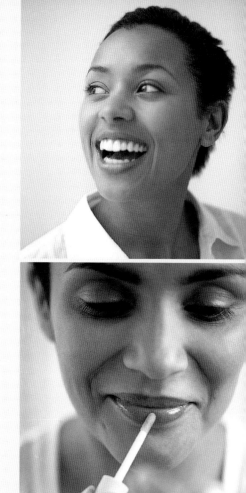

emotional acupressure

EMOTIONAL FREEDOM TECHNIQUE may sound away with the fairies, but it really works. Try it (locked in the toilet!) when you need stress relief during a difficult day. It looks complicated written down, but is very simple. Just two rounds of tapping (about 90 seconds) can shift a negative feeling.

1 First, identify and let yourself experience the uncomfortable feeling, saying it softly to yourself ('I feel scared') as you tap.

2 Start tapping the chopping edge of your right hand with the three middle fingers of your left hand.

3 Now, using the index and middle fingers of your right hand start tapping the following acupressure points on your face:
* the inner edge of the right eyebrow
* just above the outer edge of the right eyebrow
* the eye socket bone below the centre of the right eye

* the centre of the upper lip just below the nose
* the centre of the crease between chin and lower lip

4 Swap to your left hand to tap:
* the outer edge of your right top rib just inside your shoulder joint
* just inside your right armpit

5 Move back to tapping the following points on your right hand with your left:
* the outer edge of the top of your thumb, then the same place on all your fingers
* the chopping edge of your hand
* between the joints of your third and little fingers

While tapping the last point, move your eyes from top to bottom, left to right, and in a big circle, without moving your head. Then hum a few bars of a tune, count from one to five, hum again and feel your brain detach from the problem. If you don't feel better, repeat the process on the other side.

stand tall
stretch

DO THIS STRETCH when you need an
energy boost to get you through the afternoon.

* Bring your feet together with toes
touching and stand as tall as possible,
with your shoulders in line with your
hips, knees and ankles. Inhale deeply
and imagine you're lifting the top
of your head away from your body
as if someone's pulling you up by an
invisible cord in the middle of your
head. Exhale and repeat five times.

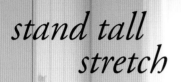

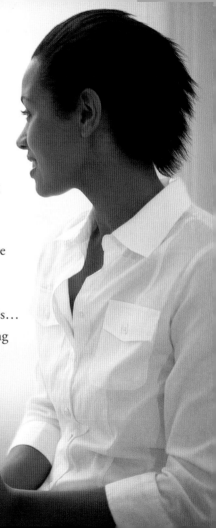

an attitude of gratitude

OUR MOOD very much depends on what we're focusing on, which means that spending a few minutes remembering what you have to be grateful for is a sure-fire way to lift your spirits. It's impossible to feel down when you're feeling grateful, so run through a checklist in your head: your friends, your partner, your children, your health, your cat, your new shoes… If life looks a little bleak right now, try focusing on the things you take for granted every day: being able to walk unaided, the freedom to choose your life, the food in your refrigerator.

5 commuter games

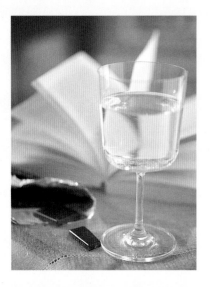

✳ See commuting as transition time from work and daydream, deep breathe or meditate to leave your 9–5 behind. Better still, walk or cycle (at least part of the way) home; exercise immediately after work not only benefits your body but releases tension, too.

✳ Meditation is simply the art of mental self-control. Whenever we focus our mind on a thought or task (even cooking a casserole), we're meditating. Choose a simple word that makes you feel good – love, peace, calm – and repeat it softly in your mind as you close your eyes. It really is that easy.

✳ Drag your mind away from day-to-day worries by forcing yourself to focus on the future. Allow

yourself to think about what you want
to be doing in a year, or two years. Not
only does this make life more exciting,
it puts short-term problems into
perspective as well.

✳ Make the most of waiting
time or delays by starting a
conversation with a fellow commuter.
Who knows what interesting
information you might pick up, and
concentrating on others is an instant
way to escape your own concerns.

✳ Imagine what you can do to
make your arrival home more
enjoyable. Dance with your children,
play with your pet, give your partner
a big hug or simply play some happy
tunes to welcome yourself home.

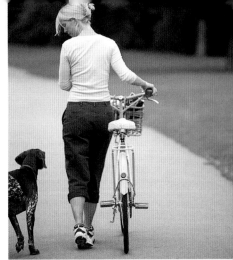

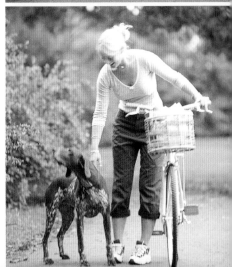

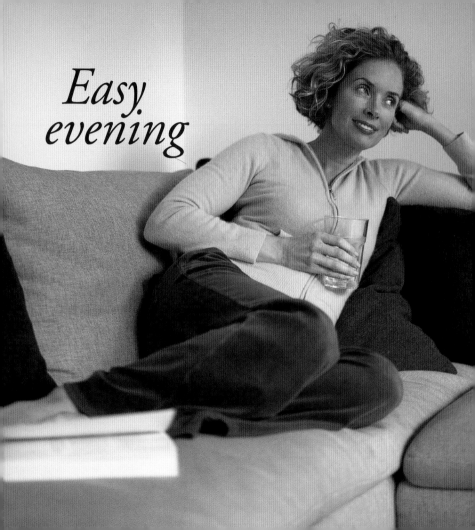

Easy.
evening

debrief your day

WRITING DOWN your thoughts is the quickest way to ease a muddled mind. By catching your feelings on paper you not only get them out of your head, but even impossible problems look so much simpler to solve. Keep a notebook or diary to record the good (a compliment) and bad (an argument), and most importantly what you felt about them. Download your day each evening and your mind will feel lighter and ready to sleep. Reread your entries regularly. Keeping a log book of your mind is the best way to discover what works for you, where you let yourself down, and what lessons are worth learning for the future.

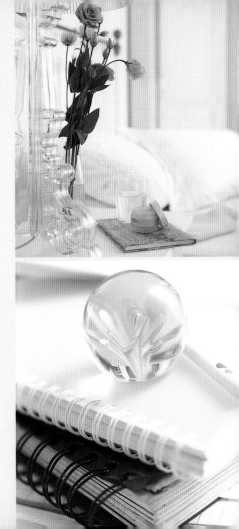

slow-down supper

THE KEY TO A RESTFUL EVENING is to calm your mind, and you can do this by eating food containing tryptophan. This amino acid helps the brain make serotonin and melatonin, neuro-transmitters that slow down your nervous system. Combine with carbohydrates (which help clear your bloodstream), and the effect will be even faster. Lighter meals will also rule out the rumblings that stop you relaxing, and don't dine after nine if you want to maximize your chance of a good night's sleep.

SNOOZE FOODS INCLUDE:
Dairy products such as cottage cheese, cheese, eggs and milk (calcium also helps the brain manufacture melatonin, so you get a double whammy); soy products; hummus; seafood; poultry; rice; wholegrains; lentils and beans; sesame and sunflower seeds; hazelnuts; and peanuts.

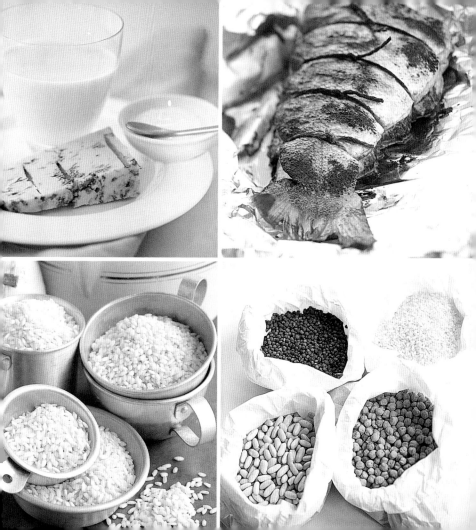

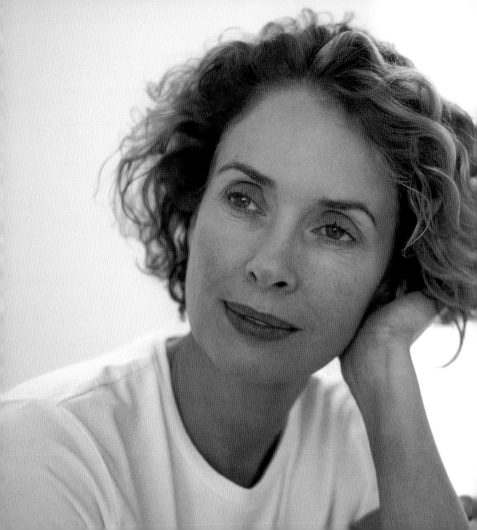

the benefits of boredom

WE'RE TAUGHT FROM CHILDHOOD that doing something (anything!) is preferable to doing nothing. But allowing yourself to relax into boredom can be very rewarding, as it gives your mind room to process your thoughts. Turn your attention inward and you'll find there's a lot going on in there. Boredom makes you realize what your worries and priorities are. Watch it without judgement and you'll experience a very comforting feeling – that your thoughts are not you, just things you're thinking. So next time you feel bored, just sit with it and let your brain bounce around until it comes to a peaceful pause.

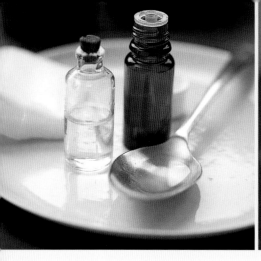
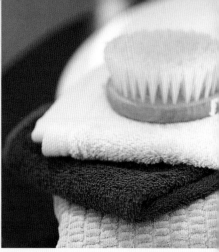

sore-muscle massage

AFTER A LONG DAY on your feet (especially if you wear high heels), these massage moves devised by Hilde Bysheim at Earthlife (see page 64) will feel like heaven.

* Rest one ankle on your opposite thigh and place both hands on your foot. With your thumbs underneath your foot, stroke upwards from heel towards toes with deep rhythmic

movements until you've covered
the whole sole of your foot.

* Support your foot with one hand
  and work on your toes. Rub,
  squeeze and gently stretch each one.

* Support your foot with one hand
  and make the other into a loose
  fist. Use your knuckles to rub
  deeply into the sole of your foot
  between the ball and the heel.

* Knead your calf muscles with
  both hands, alternating between
  squeezing and releasing the muscle
  away from the bone. Then gently
  stroke up the back of your leg with
  one hand following the other.

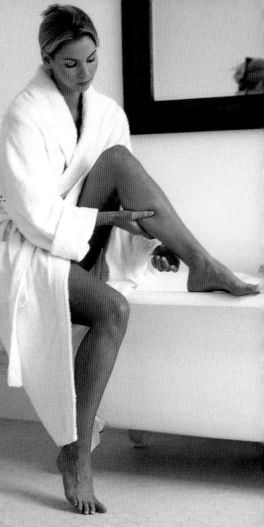

5 ways from moody to mellow

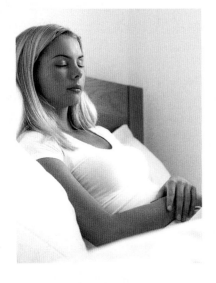

✳ Look up and you'll immediately feel uplifted. When we're low, we walk with hunched shoulders and downcast eyes, but look up and you're guaranteed to feel different.

✳ Try this simple relaxation technique after a tense day. Sit comfortably with your eyes closed. Beginning at the top of your head, scan your body for stress and gently tell it to relax ('temples relax, jaw relax, neck relax, shoulders relax' and so on). Breathe in as you say the words and out as you release the tension.

✳ The most common side effect of watching TV is mild depression, possibly because it reminds us of what we haven't got (a designer wardrobe, a perfect relationship). So rather than reaching for the remote, pick an item from your happiness hit list (see page 29) to fill your precious evening.

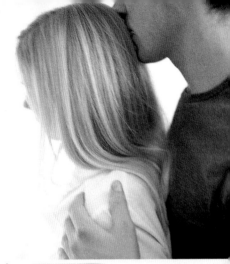

✳ Scientists have proved what we knew all along, that kissing makes us feel happier. Whether it's because we feel loved or simply that it feels so good, it's definitely worth scheduling in some affection time with your partner or children after a hard day.

✳ Being told you're loved is up there with the best of life experiences, but it also works the other way round. Expressing love for others makes us feel good too, so tell someone you care about exactly what it is that makes you love them so much.

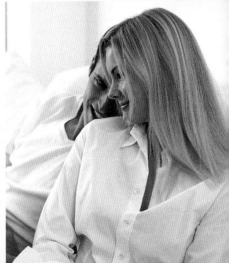

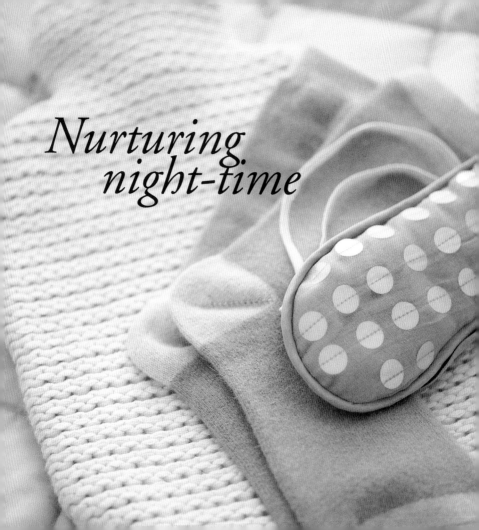

*Nurturing
night-time*

quieten the volume

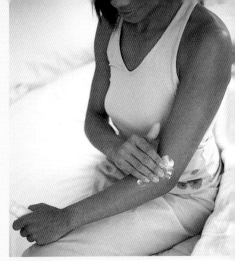

THE CURE FOR NOISE is silence. Imagine there's a control knob in your head that allows you to turn down the volume of the voices chattering away inside. Then experiment by playing around with the knob, mentally turning it up and then way down. Practise at night when the world is quiet, but also when you're surrounded by noise during the day. You may experience true quiet for the very first time. Or simply close your eyes and make a 'ssshhh' sound as though you're trying to lull a baby to sleep. It will have the same effect on your noisy brain.

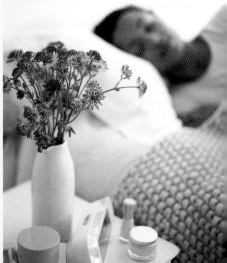

home-made bath soaks

STAY SUBMERGED for at least 10 minutes to feel
the benefits.

* Milk is both soothing and moisturizing, making it
  the perfect spa-type soak. Mix one cup of milk
  with one teaspoon of sweet almond oil and pour
  into a warm bath. Or mix two cups of milk with a
  quarter-cup of clear honey, pour into a half-filled
  bath and swish to mix before topping up the water.

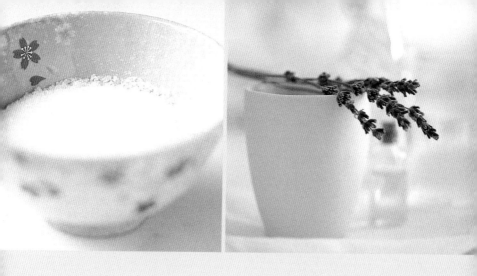

* Oatmeal soothes sensitive skin. Place one tablespoon of finely ground oats in a muslin square or the toe end of an old pair of tights, add five drops of lavender essential oil, secure, and tie to the warm tap as you run the bath. You can also rub the soaked bundle over your skin for a gentle scrub.

* Honey is naturally anti-bacterial, and so perfect for problem skin. Pour two tablespoons of honey into the running water, then add five drops of lavender oil before stepping in.

TOUCH IS ESSENTIAL to both your body and mind. When you hurt you instinctively rub it better, consciously because it acts as a local anaesthetic, but also because touch stimulates your brain into releasing endorphin-like feel-good chemicals. Without constant touch we risk becoming depressed and aggressive, and touch is also the highly addictive glue that bonds couples together. Boost your libido by keeping sex special – romantic music, candlelight, sexy nightwear – and it will never lose its appeal. And don't limit touch to twosomes. Something as simple as a neck massage has been found to reduce depression, lower stress levels and improve your quality of sleep. Try this simple technique.

the pleasure of touch

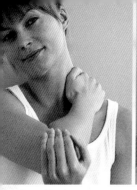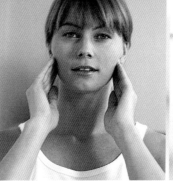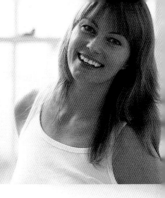

* Place your hand over your opposite shoulder and begin squeezing your flesh between thumb and fingers, supporting your elbow with the opposite hand. Repeat on the other side.

* Work from each shoulder up towards your hairline, using your fingers and thumb in small circles to find tight muscles. These will feel like thick spots or bands of tension. Apply pressure, gently but firmly, to slowly work them out.

* Using both hands, make gentle small circles up your neck either side of your spine until you reach the base of your skull.

* Hug yourself and feel around your shoulder blades for knots of tension, working up and down with your fingertips.

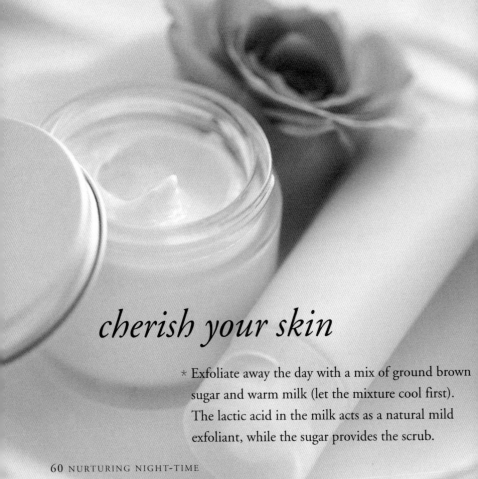

cherish your skin

* Exfoliate away the day with a mix of ground brown
sugar and warm milk (let the mixture cool first).
The lactic acid in the milk acts as a natural mild
exfoliant, while the sugar provides the scrub.

* For a luxurious (and anti-ageing) treat on dry skin, pierce a vitamin E capsule, squeeze out the contents and massage onto your face and neck.

* To loosen blackheads, combine equal parts of baking soda and water in your hand and rub gently onto your skin for 2–3 minutes before rinsing with warm water.

* To exfoliate dry lips, massage on a dab of honey mixed with a little sugar and then wipe (or lick!) off.

* Reduce swelling on tired eyes with moistened green tea bags (the polyphenols in green tea are anti-inflammatory), popped in the fridge for a few minutes.

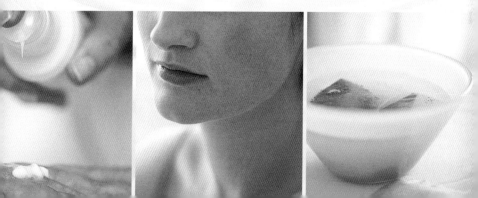

5 thoughts
to end
your day

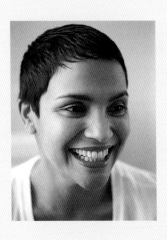

* If you can't switch off, try a little replacement thinking. Replace a worrying thought (tomorrow's meeting) with a positive one (where to go on holiday) and your mood will change.

* Adopt a selective memory. Choose to remember the best from your past, and the good feelings won't be far behind. This isn't about avoiding responsibility for your actions, it's about not filling your thoughts with unhelpful and painful memories.

* Don't worry if you can't find the solution to a problem. Now may simply not be the right time. Doing nothing may be difficult, but sometimes it's the wisest choice. When we're faced with a crisis our natural instinct is to take

control, but the situation may still be ongoing, and you'll know what to do when the time comes.

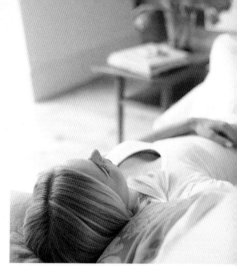

✳ Why are you alive? Having meaning in your life makes all the difference, and it's easier than you think. Create your own mission statement that sums up what you want from life ('to be surrounded by people I love', 'to experience new things') and remind yourself of it daily.

✳ Designate your head a happy space and let imagination be your salvation. Recall happy times, hum your favourite tune, look at a beautiful view. Most of us are so good at dwelling on problems that we don't realize we can choose what we think about.

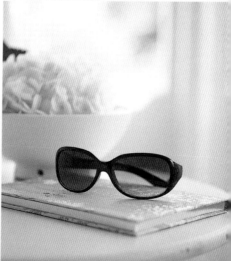

Directory

ESSENTIAL OILS
Neal's Yard Remedies
Mail order on 0845 2623145
www.nealsyardremedies.com

HOME-MADE RECIPES
*The Naturewatch Handbook
of Home-made Toiletries* is
£2.50 inc p&p by cheque to
Naturewatch
14 Hewlett Road
Cheltenham GL52 6AA
Ring 01242 252871 or
visit www.naturewatch.org
to order.

MASSAGE
Hilde Bysheim
Earthlife
Arch 2, Kew Bridge Arches
Richmond
Surrey TW9 3AW
020 8940 0888
www.earth-life.co.uk

HAIR
Steven Goldsworthy at
Goldsworthy's Hairdressing,
1 Catherine Street
Swindon SN15 5RN
01793 523817

SKINCARE
Gatineau mail order on
0800 7315805 or online
at www.thebeautyroom.com.

FITNESS
Gaiam home fitness
equipment is available in
health and department
stores. Order direct on
0870 2415471
or online at
www.gaiamdirect.co.uk.

Picture credits